THE

ULTIMATE

GUIDE TO

INTERMITTENT

FASTING FOR

BEGINNERS

—·—

UNLOCK THE POWER OF FASTING FOR OPTIMAL HEALTH AND WEIGHT LOSS

CONTENTS

1. Introduction   1
   What Is Intermittent Fasting?
   The Origins Behind Intermittent Fasting
   Overview of the Different Intermittent Fasting Methods
   Purpose and Goals of the Book

2. The Science Behind Intermittent Fasting   6
   How Intermittent Fasting Affects the Body?
   Why Insulin and Metabolism Are so Crucial in Intermittent Fasting?
   The Different Metabolic States
   How Research Studies Back Up the Efficiency of Intermittent Fasting?

3. Benefits of Intermittent Fasting   14
   Intermittent Fasting is Accessible to Everyone
   Weight Loss and Body Composition Improvements
   Unlocking the Secrets of Better Blood Sugar Control
   Eating for Health and Longevity
   Mastering Mental Clarity

Gut Feeling: A Journey to Optimal Digestive Wellness

Patience Pays Off: The Timeframe for Seeing Results with Intermittent Fasting

4. Getting Started With Intermittent Fasting   25

Unlock Your Inner Champion With This Step-By-Step Preparation

7 Tips for Success in Intermittent Fasting

Busting Myths and Overcoming Obstacles in Intermittent Fasting

Understand Your Metabolic Profile

5. Different Methods of Intermittent Fasting   36

The 16 Hour Transformation

The Two-Day Wonder Diet

The One-Day On, One-Day Off Method

Eat-Stop-Eat

6. Combining Intermittent Fasting With a Healthy Diet   48

Fuel Your Fast: The Ultimate Intermittent Fasting Food List

Maximise Your Intermittent Fasting Success With Hydration

Boost Intermittent Fasting With Supplements and Vitamins

5 Surprising Tips for a Perfect Blend of Intermittent Fasting and a Balanced Diet

Fueling Your Body Right: The Importance of Your First Meal After Intermittent Fasting

What You Should Avoid on Your Intermittent Fasting Journey

Know Your Optimal Calories Intake

7. Intermittent Fasting as a Tool for Weight Loss   72

The Importance of Weight Loss in Health

Scientific Research on Intermittent Fasting and Weight Loss

Most Effective Types of Intermittent Fasting for Weight Loss

Weight Loss Plateaus During Intermittent Fasting

Fasting for Weight Loss: How Long Does It Take to See Results?

8. Intermittent Fasting for Different Populations   82

Intermittent Fasting for Women

Women Over 50

Intermittent Fasting for Men

Athletes and Active Individuals

Muscle Gains

9. Intermittent Fasting for Risk Populations   90

Pregnant and Breastfeeding Women

Intermittent Fasting for Children

Intermittent Fasting for Individuals With Medical Conditions

10. 20 Mouth-Watering Meal Ideas to Elevate Your   100
     Intermittent Fasting Experience

11. Conclusion   111
        Special Bonus

1

— • —

INTRODUCTION

What Is Intermittent Fasting?

Intermittent Fasting is defined as a pattern of eating that alternate between periods of Fasting and eating. It is a method of calorie restriction that does not specify what foods to eat or avoid but instead focuses on when to eat. The concept is simple - by reducing the overall number of calories consumed, the body enters a state of a calorie deficit and begins to burn stored fat for energy. It has gained popularity recently as a weight loss and health-promoting technique, with a range of different Fasting styles and approaches available for individuals.

The Origins Behind Intermittent Fasting

The practice of Intermittent Fasting has a long and rich history, with evidence of its use dating back thousands of years. Throughout history, Intermittent Fasting has been used for religious, cultural, and health purposes.

In ancient civilizations such as Greece and Rome, Intermittent Fasting was used as a way to purify the body and mind and as a way to improve overall health. In religious communities, Intermittent Fasting was and still is used to show devotion and practice self-discipline.

In the early 20th century, Intermittent Fasting was popularized to improve health and prevent disease. In the mid-20th century, it was widely used to treat obesity and related health conditions.

In recent years, Intermittent Fasting has gained popularity as a weight loss and health-promoting technique, with numerous studies and clinical trials conducted to explore its potential benefits. The rise of the Intermittent Fasting movement has led to various styles and approaches, making it accessible and adaptable for individuals of all backgrounds and lifestyles.

Despite its long history, Intermittent Fasting is still a relatively new concept in the modern world, and more research is needed to understand its effects on the human body fully. Nevertheless, its popularity continues to grow, and it is widely recognized as a safe and effective way to improve overall health and promote weight loss.

Overview of the Different Intermittent Fasting Methods

Intermittent Fasting involves alternating periods of fasting with periods of eating, intending to reduce the overall number of calories consumed. There are several different methods of Intermittent Fasting, each with its own unique set of rules and guidelines.

One of the most popular Intermittent Fasting methods is the 16/8 Method. This method involves fasting for 16 hours and eating within an 8-hour window. This method is the most flexible and easy to incorporate into any lifestyle.

Another popular Intermittent Fasting method is the 5:2 Diet. This method involves eating normally for 5 days a week and restricting calories to 500-600 for the other 2 days. This method can be more challenging for some individuals but is effective for weight loss.

Alternate Day Fasting is another Intermittent Fasting method that involves fasting every other day, either by completely abstaining from food or restricting calories to 500-600. This method is more intense and may not be suitable for everyone.

In addition to these more traditional Intermittent Fasting methods, there are also a variety of other approaches, including Time-Restricted Feeding, the Warrior Diet, and the Eat-Stop-Eat method. Each method involves a unique set of rules and guidelines and may be more suitable for specific individuals based on their lifestyle, goals, and health status.

Regardless of the method chosen, Intermittent Fasting has been shown to have numerous health benefits, including weight loss, improved insulin sensitivity, decreased inflammation, and improved cardiovascular health. However, it is important to consult with a healthcare provider before starting any Intermittent Fasting method, particularly for individuals with underlying health conditions or who are taking medications.

Purpose and Goals of the Book

This book aims to provide a comprehensive and in-depth understanding of Intermittent Fasting, including its history, benefits, methods, and tips for successful implementation. This book seeks to educate and inform individuals about Intermittent Fasting and help them decide whether this approach is right for them.

Additionally, the book may aim to provide practical and actionable advice for individuals looking to incorporate Intermittent Fasting into their lives, including tips for overcoming common challenges, choosing the suitable method, and maintaining a healthy and balanced approach to eating.

Ultimately, this book aims to promote Intermittent Fasting as a safe and effective way to improve overall health and well-being and to empower individuals to make positive changes in their lives.

2

---•---

THE SCIENCE BEHIND INTERMITTENT FASTING

How Intermittent Fasting Affects the Body?

Intermittent Fasting is a practice that involves alternating periods of fasting with periods of eating. This approach to eating has been shown to have several positive effects on the body, including improved metabolism, increased weight loss, and reduced risk of chronic diseases.

One of the critical ways that Intermittent Fasting affects the body is by promoting cellular repair and rejuvenation. During Fasting, the body shifts from digestion and nutrient absorption to repairing and regenerating damaged cells. This process, known as autophagy, helps to maintain the health of the body's cells and reduce the risk of chronic diseases such as cancer, Alzheimer's, and Parkinson's.

Another meaningful way that Intermittent Fasting affects the body is through its impact on metabolism. For example, Fasting has been shown to increase insulin sensitivity, which is essential for maintaining healthy blood sugar levels and reducing the risk of type 2 diabetes. Additionally, Intermittent Fasting has been shown to increase the production of human growth hormone (HGH), which helps to boost metabolism and promote fat loss.

Intermittent Fasting has also been shown to positively impact heart health, reducing the risk of cardiovascular disease and improving markers of cardiovascular health such as cholesterol levels and blood pressure. This is partly because Intermittent Fasting has been shown to reduce inflammation, which is a crucial factor in the development of cardiovascular disease.

Finally, Intermittent Fasting has been shown to improve brain function and mental health. Fasting has been shown to increase the production of brain-derived neurotrophic factors (BDNF). This protein is essential for the growth and survival of nerve cells in the brain. This increased production of BDNF has been linked to improved cognitive function, reduced risk of depression and anxiety, and improved memory and learning ability.

Why Insulin and Metabolism Are so Crucial in Intermittent Fasting?

Insulin and metabolism play a crucial role in Intermittent Fasting and its impact on the body. Insulin is a hormone the pancreas produces that regulates blood sugar levels by helping the body store excess glucose as fat. In a typical Western diet, insulin levels are frequently elevated due to the high intake of refined carbohydrates and sugar.

During Intermittent Fasting, insulin levels naturally decrease as the body shifts from a state of digestion to a state of repair and rejuvenation. This decrease in insulin levels allows the body to access and burn stored fat for energy, leading to weight loss and improved insulin sensitivity.

Improved insulin sensitivity is a key aspect of Intermittent Fasting and its impact on metabolism. Insulin sensitivity refers to the body's ability to respond to insulin and regulate blood sugar levels. In individuals with poor insulin sensitivity, insulin levels remain elevated, increasing fat storage and risk of type 2 diabetes.

Intermittent Fasting has been shown to increase insulin sensitivity, which can help to improve overall metabolic health and reduce the risk of chronic diseases such as type 2 diabetes and cardiovascular disease. Additionally, Intermittent Fasting has been shown to increase the production of human growth hormone (HGH), which helps to boost metabolism and promote fat loss.

Intermittent Fasting also has a positive impact on the regulation of glucose and insulin, leading to improved blood sugar control. In addition, by reducing insulin levels, Intermittent Fasting can help to enhance the body's ability to access and burn stored fat for energy, leading to weight loss and improved metabolic health.

In conclusion, insulin and metabolism play a crucial role in Intermittent Fasting and its impact on the body. By reducing insulin levels and improving insulin sensitivity, Intermittent Fasting can help to improve overall metabolic health, reduce the risk of chronic diseases, and promote weight loss. By incorporating Intermittent Fasting into your life, you can help to maintain and improve your overall health and well-being.

The Different Metabolic States

Intermittent Fasting involves alternating periods of Fasting and eating, which triggers changes in the body and elicits different metabolic states. These metabolic states are crucial for optimizing health benefits. Understanding them is critical to successfully incorporating Intermittent Fasting into your routine.

The first metabolic state that occurs during Intermittent Fasting is the fed state. The fed state occurs during the eating period and lasts several hours after a meal. During the fed state, insulin levels are elevated, and the body is focused on digestion, absorption, and storage of nutrients. In this state, the body is not in fat-burning mode, as insulin signals the body to store excess energy as fat.

The second metabolic state is the post-absorptive state, which occurs after the fed state has ended and the body is no longer in a state of digestion. In this state, insulin levels drop, and the body shifts into a state of repair and rejuvenation. During the post-absorptive state, the body begins to break down stored glycogen for energy and accesses stored fat as a secondary energy source. This is the fat-burning state, and it is in this state that the body can reap the benefits of Intermittent Fasting, including weight loss and improved metabolic health.

The third metabolic state is the starved state, which occurs after several hours of Fasting. In the starved state, insulin levels remain low, and the body continues to access stored fat for energy. In this state, the body begins to produce ketones, which are a by-product of fat breakdown and can be used for energy. This is the state in which the body reaches ketosis. In this state, the benefits of Intermittent Fasting are most pronounced, including improved insulin sensitivity, reduced inflammation, and improved cognitive function.

Intermittent Fasting elicits changes in the body that trigger different metabolic states, each with its own unique benefits. Understanding these metabolic states is crucial to incorporating Intermittent Fasting into your routine and maximizing its benefits. By understanding the different metabolic conditions and how Intermittent Fasting affects the body, you can make informed decisions about incorporating Intermittent Fasting into your life for optimal health and well-being.

How Research Studies Back Up the Efficiency of Intermittent Fasting?

Intermittent Fasting has gained popularity in recent years to improve health and well-being. However, many people are sceptical about its effectiveness and want solid scientific evidence to support its claims. Fortunately, many research studies have been conducted on Intermittent Fasting that has provided insight into its effects on the body and its potential benefits.

One of the most well-known studies on Intermittent Fasting was conducted by Dr Jason Fung, a leading expert in Intermittent Fasting. In his study, Dr Fung found that Intermittent Fasting led to significant weight loss, improved insulin sensitivity, and reduced inflammation in obese individuals. This study was published in the International Journal of Obesity. It demonstrated the potential benefits of Intermittent Fasting for weight management and metabolic health.

Another study by researchers at the University of Illinois found that Intermittent Fasting led to improved insulin sensitivity and reduced inflammation in obese individuals. This study was published in the Journal of Nutritional Biochemistry. It provided further support for the benefits of Intermittent Fasting for metabolic health.

Furthermore, a study conducted by researchers at the University of California, Los Angeles, found that Intermittent Fasting led to improved cognitive function and reduced oxidative stress in mice. This study was published in the journal Age and provides evidence for the potential benefits of Intermittent Fasting for brain health.

These are just a few examples of the many research studies conducted on Intermittent Fasting. The results of these studies provide strong evidence for the effectiveness of Intermittent Fasting and its potential benefits for health and well-being.

It is important to note that while Intermittent Fasting is effective in numerous studies, more research is needed to fully understand its effects on the body and its long-term benefits. Additionally, Intermittent Fasting may only be suitable for some. Individuals should speak with their healthcare provider before starting an Intermittent Fasting program to determine if it is right for them.

In conclusion, Intermittent Fasting has been shown to be effective in numerous research studies, with potential benefits for weight management, metabolic health, brain health, and overall well-being. While more research is needed to understand its effects fully, the results of existing studies provide strong evidence for the effectiveness of Intermittent Fasting as a tool for improving health and well-being.

3

— • —

BENEFITS OF INTERMITTENT FASTING

Intermittent Fasting is Accessible to Everyone

One of the most appealing aspects of this approach is its accessibility. Unlike many other health and wellness strategies that can be expensive or require significant lifestyle changes, intermittent fasting is simple, free, and flexible. This makes it accessible to everyone.

The idea of intermittent fasting is simple. Unlike other diets that require complex calculations and meal planning, intermittent fasting only requires you to adjust the timing of your meals. By limiting your eating window to a set number of hours per day or week, you can achieve many of the same benefits as more complicated diets. This simplicity makes intermittent fasting easy to follow and incorporate into your daily routine.

Secondly, intermittent fasting is free. You don't need special equipment or expensive memberships to get started. All you need is a willingness to adjust your eating schedule and stick to your chosen fasting method. This affordability means that anyone can try intermittent fasting, regardless of their financial situation.

Finally, intermittent fasting is flexible. There are many different methods to choose from, so you can find one that works best for your lifestyle and preferences. Whether you prefer a daily eating window or a more extended fast a few times a week, there is an intermittent fasting method that will work for you. This flexibility means that you can adjust your fasting schedule to fit your schedule, making it a sustainable long-term approach to health and wellness.

Weight Loss and Body Composition Improvements

Intermittent fasting can lead to significant weight loss and body composition improvements, as the body is forced to burn stored fat and sugar to produce energy. This results in the reduction of body fat and can lead to a leaner appearance.

Individuals who engage in intermittent fasting may experience a decrease in body weight, reduced waist circumference, lower body fat percentage, and an increase in lean muscle mass. These changes can help improve overall body composition, leading to a healthier, more toned appearance.

Intermittent fasting has also been shown to improve insulin sensitivity, which can help regulate glucose levels and prevent the accumulation of fat in the body. This can lead to a reduction in the risk of obesity and related health problems such as type 2 diabetes, heart disease, and certain cancers.

Additionally, intermittent fasting can have a positive impact on overall health, as the body is given the time and space to focus on repairing and regenerating cells. This can lead to an increase in energy levels, better sleep patterns, and an overall improvement in mood and mental well-being.

It is important to note that while the effects of intermittent fasting on weight loss and body composition are promising, individual results may vary. Further research is needed to fully understand the impact of different types of intermittent fasting methods on weight loss and body composition.

Unlocking the Secrets of Better Blood Sugar Control

Intermittent fasting has been shown to have a positive impact on insulin sensitivity, which is the ability of the body to respond effectively to insulin and regulate glucose levels. This can lead to numerous health benefits and a reduced risk of certain diseases.

When insulin sensitivity is improved, the body is better able to control glucose levels, reducing the risk of developing type 2 diabetes. This is because insulin can regulate the uptake of glucose into the cells more effectively, preventing excess glucose from being stored as fat.

Intermittent fasting can also have a positive impact on the metabolism, increasing the rate at which the body burns calories. This can lead to an improvement in overall body composition, with a reduction in body fat and an increase in lean muscle mass.

Additionally, improved insulin sensitivity can have a positive impact on overall health, leading to an increase in energy levels, better sleep patterns, and a reduction in the risk of heart disease and certain cancers.

Intermittent fasting has also been shown to increase the production of human growth hormone (HGH), which has numerous health benefits, including increased insulin sensitivity, improved bone density, and a reduction in the risk of certain diseases.

Eating for Health and Longevity

Intermittent fasting has been linked to increased longevity and a reduced risk of chronic diseases. The underlying mechanisms behind these benefits are complex, and involve a range of physiological changes that occur in response to fasting.

One of the key benefits of intermittent fasting is its impact on the body's oxidative stress levels. Oxidative stress occurs when the body's antioxidant defense mechanisms are overwhelmed by free radicals, leading to cellular damage and an increased risk of disease. Intermittent fasting has been shown to reduce oxidative stress levels, helping to protect cells and reduce the risk of chronic diseases.

Intermittent fasting has also been linked to improved cellular and molecular processes. This includes the activation of certain genetic pathways that have been linked to increased longevity, such as the sirtuin pathway. Additionally, intermittent fasting has been shown to improve the efficiency of the body's energy-producing processes, increasing energy levels and overall health.

Another key benefit of intermittent fasting is its impact on the immune system. Intermittent fasting has been shown to increase the production of immune cells, helping to protect against infections and chronic diseases. Additionally, intermittent fasting has been linked to reduced inflammation, a key factor in the development of many chronic diseases.

Intermittent fasting has also been linked to a reduction in the risk of several chronic diseases, including type 2 diabetes, cardiovascular disease, and certain cancers. This is due in part to its impact on insulin sensitivity and glucose regulation, which help to reduce the risk of these diseases.

Mastering Mental Clarity

Intermittent fasting has been shown to have a positive impact on mental clarity and focus. The human brain requires energy in order to function, and this energy comes from glucose, which is derived from carbohydrates in the diet. Intermittent fasting restricts calorie intake for a certain period of time, reducing the amount of glucose available for the brain to use. This reduction in glucose stimulates the production of alternative sources of fuel for the brain, such as ketones.

Ketones are produced when the body breaks down fat stores for energy, and they have been shown to provide a more efficient and sustainable source of energy for the brain than glucose. The brain's increased reliance on ketones as a source of fuel during intermittent fasting may improve mental clarity and focus.

In addition, intermittent fasting has been shown to increase the production of brain-derived neurotrophic factor (BDNF), a protein that plays a key role in the growth, maturation, and survival of neurons in the brain. Higher levels of BDNF have been linked to improved cognitive function, reduced symptoms of depression, and reduced risk of age-related cognitive decline.

Intermittent fasting may also reduce oxidative stress and inflammation in the brain, which have been linked to a range of neurological disorders, including Alzheimer's disease, Parkinson's disease, and multiple sclerosis. By reducing oxidative stress and inflammation, intermittent fasting may help to protect and preserve brain function, leading to improved mental clarity and focus.

It is important to note that the effects of intermittent fasting on mental clarity and focus may vary between individuals and may depend on factors such as the duration and frequency of fasting periods, the individual's baseline level of cognitive function, and the presence of underlying health conditions.

Gut Feeling: A Journey to Optimal Digestive Wellness

Intermittent fasting has been shown to have a positive impact on digestion and gut health. This is largely due to the fact that fasting allows the digestive system to take a break and reset, which can be beneficial for people who struggle with digestive issues.

Fasting can improve the balance of gut bacteria, which is crucial for overall digestive health. A growing body of research has shown that an imbalance in gut bacteria can lead to a number of health problems, including digestive issues, allergies, and autoimmune diseases. Intermittent fasting can help to improve this balance by promoting the growth of beneficial bacteria and reducing the populations of harmful bacteria.

Intermittent fasting can also reduce inflammation in the gut, which can lead to improved digestion and reduced symptoms of digestive disorders such as irritable bowel syndrome (IBS) and Crohn's disease. Inflammation in the gut can cause a number of digestive issues, including pain, bloating, and diarrhea. By reducing inflammation, intermittent fasting can help to alleviate these symptoms and improve overall gut health.

In addition, fasting has been shown to improve gut motility, which can help to promote regular bowel movements and reduce symptoms of constipation. This can be particularly beneficial for people who struggle with digestive issues, as regular bowel movements are crucial for maintaining good gut health.

Another way that intermittent fasting can benefit digestion is by promoting the production of digestive enzymes. These enzymes help to break down food in the stomach and intestines, which can make it easier for the body to absorb nutrients. By promoting the production of digestive enzymes, intermittent fasting can help to improve the overall efficiency of the digestive system.

Patience Pays Off: The Timeframe for Seeing Results with Intermittent Fasting

One of the most common questions people have when starting intermittent fasting is, "How long will it take to see results?" The answer is that it varies from person to person, but typically it takes between 6 to 8 weeks to fully feel the effects of intermittent fasting.

During the first few weeks of intermittent fasting, many people experience a decrease in hunger and an increase in energy levels. However, it can take some time for the body to adjust to the new eating pattern and fully realize the benefits.

The type of intermittent fasting that someone chooses to follow also has an impact on the timeframe for seeing results. For instance, the 16/8 method may result in more immediate changes than the 5:2 diet or alternate day fasting. This is due to the fact that the 16/8 method has a shorter fasting window, which may be more manageable for some individuals. Since the body is not deprived of nutrients for an extended period, it may respond more quickly to this type of fasting.

On the other hand, the 5:2 diet or alternate day fasting may require a longer timeframe to see noticeable results. With these methods, there are days where the body is undergoing a more prolonged period of fasting, which may take more time for the body to adapt to. However, once the body becomes accustomed to the fasting schedule, individuals may experience significant health benefits. Tips and information will be provided over the book.

Additionally, it's important to consider other factors that may impact the timeframe for seeing results. For example, someone who is already following a healthy diet and exercise routine may see results sooner than someone who is just starting to make lifestyle changes.

4

— · —

GETTING STARTED WITH INTERMITTENT FASTING

Unlock Your Inner Champion With This Step-By-Step Preparation

Congratulations on making the decision to unlock your inner champ with intermittent fasting! This powerful diet trend has taken the world by storm, with countless people experiencing weight loss, improved digestion, and increased energy levels. However, before diving in, it's essential to take the time to properly prepare yourself for success.

The first step in preparing for intermittent fasting is to consult with a healthcare professional. They can help you determine if this diet is safe for you, provide guidance on making any necessary adjustments, and ensure that you're on the right track to achieving your health goals.

Next, look honestly at your current eating habits and food choices. Are you consuming too much processed or junk food? Do you struggle with overeating? Identifying areas where you can make healthier choices and improve your nutrition will be crucial to your success with intermittent fasting.

Transitioning to intermittent fasting may take some time, primarily if you're used to regularly eating throughout the day. Start by reducing the number of meals you eat each day and gradually increasing your fasting periods. This will help your body adjust to the new eating pattern and prevent unpleasant side effects.

To stay on track with your fasting goals, it's essential to plan your meals in advance. Focus on eating nutritious, balanced meals during your eating periods, and avoid processed and junk foods, which can sabotage your efforts and leave you feeling sluggish and unwell.

Managing stress levels is also a critical component of successful intermittent fasting. Stress can wreak havoc on your health, making it more challenging to adhere to your fasting schedule. Incorporating stress management techniques, such as mindfulness and exercise, into your daily routine will help you stay focused and motivated.

Remember, your body is unique; what works for one person may not work for you. Be patient and listen to your body, making any necessary adjustments to your fasting schedule based on your needs and health status. Finally, celebrate your progress and stay committed to your goals. You'll be well on your way to unlocking your inner champion with intermittent fasting!

7 Tips for Success in Intermittent Fasting

Intermittent fasting is a popular dietary approach that involves alternating periods of eating with periods of fasting. While this approach can be practical for weight loss and improving overall health, it can also be challenging. However, with the right tips and strategies, anyone can succeed with intermittent fasting. This chapter will explore practical and actionable advice to help you get the most out of your fasting journey and reach your health and wellness goals. Whether you're a seasoned pro or just starting out, these tips will give you the confidence and guidance you need to succeed. So let's dive in and get started!

1. Stick to your schedule: Choose a fasting schedule that works best for you and stick to it as consistently as possible. This will help you better regulate your body's hunger cues and smooth the transition to intermittent fasting.

2. Plan your meals: Plan your meals in advance and focus on eating nutritious, balanced meals during your eating periods. Avoid

processed and junk foods and focus on eating plenty of fruits, vegetables, lean protein, and healthy fats.

3. Stay hydrated: Drinking plenty of water during fasting is essential to avoid dehydration and help flush out toxins from your body. You can also drink calorie-free beverages, such as herbal tea or water infused with fruit, to help keep you hydrated and satisfied.

4. Exercise regularly: Exercise can help improve insulin sensitivity and boost weight loss, making it an essential component of an intermittent fasting regimen. Aim for at least 30 minutes of moderate exercise daily, such as brisk walking or cycling.

5. Get enough sleep: Getting enough sleep is essential for good health and can help you better manage the effects of intermittent fasting. Aim for 7-9 hours of sleep each night.

6. Manage stress levels: Stress can have a negative impact on your health and may make it more challenging to stick to your fasting schedule. Make sure to incorporate stress management techniques like mindfulness and exercise into your routine.

7. Be mindful of your hunger cues: Listen to your body and pay attention to your hunger cues. For example, if you're starving during fasting, try to drink more water or engage in physical activity to help manage your hunger.

In conclusion, incorporating tips for success in intermittent fasting can help maximize the benefits of this dietary approach and make the experience more manageable. Whether preparing ahead of time, finding the proper eating schedule that works for you, or staying hydrated, incorporating these tips can help support a successful and sustainable journey with intermittent fasting.

As an added bonus to the seven tips for success in intermittent fasting, we recommend trying Yogaburn. This ultimate online yoga program complements your fasting routine while providing many benefits for your mind and body. By incorporating Yogaburn into your intermittent fasting journey, you'll enhance your weight loss goals and improve your focus, mentality, and overall well-being. So don't miss this extra bonus - sign up for Yogaburn today!

Busting Myths and Overcoming Obstacles in Intermittent Fasting

Intermittent fasting has become a buzzword in the world of health and fitness, promising weight loss, improved energy, and various other benefits. However, like with any new lifestyle change, several myths and obstacles can make it challenging to stick to this diet. As an author and health enthusiast, I want to debunk some of these misconceptions and provide practical tips to help you successfully implement intermittent fasting into your lifestyle.

One of the most common misconceptions about intermittent fasting is that it triggers the body to go into "starvation mode." This mode is thought to slow down the metabolism, making it harder to lose weight. However, this is not the case with intermittent fasting. Unlike prolonged fasting, intermittent fasting allows for adequate caloric intake during eating. Therefore, your body is less nutrient-deprived and less likely to go into starvation mode.

Another challenge people often face when starting intermittent fasting is a lack of energy. This can be incredibly daunting at the beginning when the body is still adjusting to the new eating pattern. To combat this, staying hydrated and engaging in physical activity to boost your energy levels is essential. When you exercise, your body releases endorphins, which can help to improve your mood and give you an extra burst of energy. Additionally, drinking plenty of water can help to keep you feeling full and reduce the likelihood of hunger pangs.

Speaking of hunger pangs, this is another challenge that many people face when implementing intermittent fasting. It's important to remember that hunger is a natural response of the body when it has gone without food for an extended period. However, there are ways to manage these pangs without breaking your fast. For example, drinking water can help to reduce hunger, and some people find that engaging in physical activity or practising mindfulness techniques, such as deep breathing or meditation, can also help to alleviate these pangs.

Another obstacle many people face when attempting intermittent fasting is difficulty sticking to a consistent schedule. This is especially true for those with a busy lifestyle or irregular work schedule. To overcome this challenge, planning your meals in advance and being mindful of your hunger cues is crucial. Preparing meals can help you consume enough nutrients and calories during your eating periods. In addition, bringing your hunger cues can help you determine when to break your fast.

Lastly, it's essential to recognize that intermittent fasting results can be inconsistent and may vary depending on individual factors such as genetics, lifestyle, and overall health status. While some people may experience rapid weight loss and improved energy, others may not see significant changes. To maximize your results, focusing on eating a healthy, balanced diet and engaging in regular physical activity is essential.

One final challenge many people face when attempting intermittent fasting is social pressure. It can be challenging to maintain this eating pattern when surrounded by friends and family who are not following the same diet. However, it's crucial to communicate your intentions to your loved ones and bring healthy snacks or beverages to social events. This way, you can still enjoy the company of your friends and family while sticking to your fasting schedule.

By understanding these common misconceptions and challenges and following the tips for overcoming them, you can successfully implement intermittent fasting into your lifestyle and achieve your health and wellness goals.

Understand Your Metabolic Profile

As you start your journey with intermittent fasting, it's important to understand your body and how it processes energy. Everyone's metabolism is unique, but we can generally categorize them into two profiles: sugar burners and fat burners.

Sugar burners rely on glucose from carbohydrates for energy, while fat burners utilize stored fat as their primary energy source. This distinction can greatly impact your intermittent fasting journey, so let's take a closer look at each profile.

Sugar burners tend to experience more frequent hunger pangs and mood swings when they don't eat regularly. They often crave sugary and starchy foods and may even experience fatigue or shakiness if they go too long without eating. This is because their body is used to constantly receiving a steady supply of glucose for energy.

On the other hand, fat burners tend to have more stable energy levels and don't experience the same intense hunger or cravings as sugar burners. Their bodies have adapted to using stored fat as fuel, which means they can go longer periods without food and still feel energized.

So, how does this impact your intermittent fasting journey?

Once you determine whether you are a sugar burner or a fat burner, you can tailor your fasting schedule and type to maximize your results. If you're a sugar burner, it may be helpful to start with a shorter fasting window and gradually work your way up to longer fasts. This will help your body become more efficient at burning fat for fuel instead of relying on glucose.

For example, if you're just starting out with intermittent fasting and you're a sugar burner, you may want to try the 12/12 method for a week or two. This method involves fasting for 12 hours and eating during a 12-hour window. Once you feel comfortable with this schedule, you can gradually increase your fasting window by an hour per day until you reach the 16/8 method and then eventually try different and more intense methods.

If you're a fat burner, you may find that you can tolerate longer fasting windows without feeling hungry or fatigued. You may also be able to handle more intense fasting schedules, such as alternate day fasting or the 5:2 diet.

Ultimately, the key is to listen to your body and adjust your fasting schedule and type as needed. It's also important to make sure you're fueling your body with nutritious foods during your eating window to support your overall health and well-being.

Remember, intermittent fasting is a journey and it may take some trial and error to find the schedule and type that works best for you.

5

— • —

DIFFERENT METHODS OF INTERMITTENT FASTING

The 16 Hour Transformation

One of the most popular fasting methods is the 16/8 method, also known as the Leangains method.

A 16/8 method involves fasting for 16 hours and eating for 8 hours. Only water, black coffee, and other non-caloric beverages are allowed during the fasting period. This feeding method is known as time-restricted feeding because it restricts the amount of food an individual consumes throughout a period.

The 16/8 method was popularized by Martin Berkhan, a Swedish fitness expert and blogger who founded the Leangains website. Berkhan developed the 16/8 method to help his clients achieve their fitness goals, and the method gained widespread popularity due to its simplicity and flexibility.

Pros:

· Increased insulin sensitivity: By restricting eating to a specific time frame, the 16/8 method can improve insulin sensitivity, which leads to better blood sugar control.

· Increased fat loss: The 16/8 method has been shown to promote weight loss, as the body burns stored fat for energy during fasting.

· Improved digestion: By giving the digestive system a break from processing food for several hours each day, the 16/8 method can improve gut health and prevent digestive problems.

· Increased mental clarity: Fasting has been shown to improve mental clarity and focus, potentially due to reduced inflammation and oxidative stress.

· Convenience: The 16/8 method is simple to follow and does not require counting calories or tracking food intake.

Cons:

· Hunger: Fasting for 16 hours can be challenging for some people, especially in the beginning. This can result in appetite, weakness, and fatigue.

· Reduced athletic performance: The 16/8 method may not be ideal for athletes or those who engage in regular physical activity, as the lack of fuel during the fasting period may affect performance.

· Social limitations: Eating during a limited time window may make it difficult to socialize with friends and family over meals, which can be challenging for some people.

· Nutrient deficiencies: If not planned carefully, the 16/8 method may result in nutrient deficiencies, as a person may not consume enough vitamins and minerals over a day.

How to start:

Begin by setting your eating window to 10-12 hours and gradually reducing it until you reach the 8-hour window. You can reduce 1 hour per day until you get the 8-hour window. You can also be creative about when you implement your eating window during the day. During fasting, drink plenty of water and incorporate low-intensity exercise to help curb hunger pangs.

In conclusion, while the 16/8 Method of intermittent fasting provides a range of benefits, it is wise to consider both the pros and cons. This is before deciding whether it is the right approach for you. It may be helpful to talk to a doctor or a nutritionist to determine the most appropriate action.

The Two-Day Wonder Diet

This 5:2 diet involves consuming a regular diet for 5 days of the week and then restricting calorie intake to 500-600 calories for 2 non-consecutive days. The 5:2 diet was popularized by Dr Michael Mosley, a British journalist and medical doctor who wrote a book on the subject in 2013.

The 5:2 diet gained popularity due to its flexibility and simplicity, as it doesn't require completely eliminating certain foods or adhering to strict eating schedules. Instead, the non-fasting days allow for standard eating patterns, making them easier to follow and adhere to in the long term.

Pros:

·   Weight loss: The 5:2 diet is effective for weight loss, as the restriction of calories for two days can reduce overall calorie intake.

·   Increased insulin sensitivity: By alternating between days of normal eating and calorie restriction, the 5:2 diet can improve insulin sensitivity and help regulate blood sugar levels.

·   Improved cardiovascular health: Studies have suggested that the 5:2 diet may improve markers of cardiovascular health, such as reducing blood pressure and cholesterol levels.

Cons:

·   Hunger: Restricting calories to 500-600 calories for two days can be challenging and may result in feelings of appetite, weakness, and fatigue.

·   Reduced athletic performance: The 5:2 diet may not be ideal for athletes or those who engage in regular physical activity, as reducing calorie intake in two days may affect performance.

·   Nutrient deficiencies: If not planned carefully, the 5:2 diet may result in nutrient deficiencies, as a person may not consume enough vitamins and minerals for a week.

·   Difficulty sticking to the diet: The 5:2 diet can be challenging to follow long-term, as it requires consistency and discipline to normally eat for five days and restrict calories for two days.

How to start:

Begin by eating normally for five days and then restrict your calories to 500-600 for the remaining two days. It's best to choose non-consecutive days for the lower calorie days, such as Tuesday and Friday. Over time, you can gradually decrease the number of calories you consume on the low-calorie days and increase the number of days per week you practice the 5:2 diet as your body becomes more accustomed to this eating pattern.

In conclusion, the 5:2 diet method in intermittent fasting allows individuals to experience the benefits of caloric restriction while still enjoying their regular meals for the majority of the week. However, it is crucial to consider one's needs and abilities before deciding if this method suits them.

The One-Day On, One-Day Off Method

The Alternate-Day Fasting Method, also known as the One-Day On, One-Day Off method is a type of intermittent fasting where individuals alternate between days of restricted calorie intake and days of normal eating. On restricted calorie intake days, individuals consume only 20-50% of their typical calorie intake. In contrast, on ordinary eating days, they usually eat.

Alternate-day fasting (ADF) has been practised for centuries, with various religious and cultural traditions promoting periodic fasting for spiritual and health benefits. Some of the earliest recorded instances of ADF date back to ancient civilizations such as Greece and Egypt, where fasting was believed to be a way of purifying the body and soul. In many religions, fasting is still a common practice and is believed to bring physical and spiritual benefits.

In modern times, ADF gained popularity in the 20th century when it was used as a weight loss method. However, it was not until the early 2000s that scientific research on ADF began to emerge. In 2003, a study conducted by researchers from the University of Illinois at Chicago found that ADF led to significant weight loss and improvements in various health markers in overweight adults.

Pros:

·   Weight Loss: This method of intermittent fasting can lead to weight loss as the overall calorie intake is reduced.

·   Increased Insulin Sensitivity: By alternating days of calorie restriction, the Alternate-Day Fasting Method may regulate blood sugar levels and improve insulin sensitivity.

·   Improved Diet Quality: On days when calorie intake is unrestricted, individuals following this method may make healthier food choices due to increased awareness and conscious decision-making.

·   Improved Mood: The changes in hormones and energy levels associated with this fasting method may lead to enhanced mood and increased mental clarity.

Cons:

·   Difficulty sticking to the plan: Alternating between days of eating normally and restricting calorie intake can be challenging, especially for those with a busy lifestyle.

· Hunger: The days of restricted calorie intake can result in feelings of hunger, making it challenging to stick to the plan.

· Reduced athletic performance: The Alternate-Day Fasting Method may not be ideal for athletes or those who engage in regular physical activity, as lowering calorie intake every other day can affect performance.

· Potentially unhealthy restriction: If not planned carefully, the Alternate-Day Fasting Method may result in restrictive and harmful eating patterns.

How to start:

Start by reducing your calorie intake on alternate days to ease into this method. For example, on your first fasting day, you can aim to consume around 500-600 calories. Then, on your non-fasting days, eat normally without overindulging. Over time, you can gradually reduce your calorie intake on fasting days and extend your fasting window.

In conclusion, The Alternate-Day Fasting Method stands out as a dynamic approach to intermittent fasting that offers a range of targeted benefits. With its carefully structured regimen alternating between days of restricted and unrestricted calorie intake, this method can help individuals achieve their weight loss goals, regulate their blood sugar levels, make healthier food choices, improve their mood and mental clarity, and boost their overall metabolic health. While it may not be suitable for everyone, the

Alternate-Day Fasting Method has the potential to revolution-
ize how individuals approach diet and health.

Eat-Stop-Eat

The 24-Hour Fasting Method, also known as "Eat-Stop-Eat",
is an intermittent fasting method that involves fasting for
24 hours once or twice a week. In this method, individuals
consume only water, black coffee, or tea for 24 hours and then
usually eat during the remaining days.

Historically, fasting has been used for various reasons, including promoting health and healing and for spiritual and
religious purposes. 24-hour fasting has been used in many
spiritual practices. It has been shown to help people feel more
connected to themselves and to a higher power.

Here are some of the pros and cons of the 24-hour fasting
method:

Pros:

·   Weight Loss: One of the primary benefits of 24-hour
fasting is weight loss. By reducing the overall number of calories

consumed, the body can enter into a metabolic state that promotes fat burning, leading to weight loss over time.

· Improved Metabolic Health: 24-hour fasting has been shown to improve insulin sensitivity and lower blood sugar levels, which can positively impact overall metabolic health.

· Increased Mental Clarity: Some people report feeling more focused and alert after a 24-hour fast, possibly due to reduced insulin levels and increased growth hormone production.

· Simplicity: Unlike many other diets and eating plans, the 24-hour fasting method is straightforward and easy to follow. All you have to do is eat for a certain period and then fast for 24 hours.

Cons:

· Hunger and Fatigue: Fasting for 24 hours can be challenging; many people report feeling hungry and fatigued during this time. This can make it difficult to stick to the fasting plan, especially for those new to fasting.

· Social Disruptions: The 24-hour fasting method may also make it challenging to participate in social activities and events that revolve around food, such as dinner parties and family gatherings.

· May not be suitable for everyone: 24-hour fasting may not be ideal for everyone, especially those with certain medical conditions such as hypoglycemia, diabetes, and other conditions that require careful monitoring of calorie and nutrient intake.

How to start:

Start with shorter fasting windows: Begin with a 12- or 16-hour fasting window, gradually increasing the fasting time by one hour per day until you're comfortable with a 24-hour fast. Also, it is essential that you choose the right day: Select a day when you can relax, avoid stressful situations, and don't have too many obligations. This will help you focus on the fast and not be distracted by other things.

In conclusion, the 24-hour fasting involves abstaining from food for 24 hours and consuming meals within a specified eating window. This form of intermittent fasting has been gaining popularity for its potential health benefits, including weight loss, improved insulin sensitivity, reduced inflammation, and increased longevity. Additionally, 24-hour fasting may help individuals develop healthier eating habits and increase mindfulness around food.

However, it's essential to proceed with caution and seek medical advice before trying 24-hour fasting, especially if you have a medical condition, pregnant, breastfeeding, or underweight. This method may not be suitable for everyone and monitoring its impact and adjusting as necessary is crucial.

Dare to try

Congratulations! You are now armed with the knowledge of four different types of intermittent fasting methods that can help you unlock the power of fasting for optimal health and weight loss.

But with so many choices, how do you choose the best method for you? The answer is simple - experiment! Find the method that suits your lifestyle and preferences, and stick to it consistently. With time, you will discover which method works best for you and reap fasting benefits. Remember, intermittent fasting is not a one-size-fits-all approach. What works for your friend or colleague may not work for you, and that's okay. Embrace intermittent fasting flexibility and be open to trying new methods until you find the perfect fit. While experimenting, pay close attention to your body and how it responds to fasting. Don't be afraid to adjust the fasting window if you experience negative effects. The goal is to find a sustainable method that works for you in the long run.

So, are you ready to take the first step towards a healthier you? Try one of the four intermittent fasting methods discussed and discover fasting's benefits for yourself. Your weight loss and health goals can be achieved with dedication and determination.

6

COMBINING INTERMITTENT FASTING WITH A HEALTHY DIET

Fuel Your Fast: The Ultimate Intermittent Fasting Food List

Intermittent fasting is a flexible diet that involves alternating periods of fasting with periods of eating, and the foods you eat during the eating periods can significantly impact the success of your fast. Choosing the right foods can help ensure that you stay full, satisfied, and energised during your fasting periods and reap the health benefits of this diet. Here are some recommended foods for intermittent fasting:

High-protein foods: Protein is essential for building and repairing muscle, supporting the immune system, and maintaining a healthy metabolism. In fact, it's often referred to as the body's building block. DurinIn addition, during Intermittent fasting, the body may be in a state of catabolism, where it breaks down muscle tissue for energy. Hence, it's crucial to consume enough protein to avoid High-protein

High protein foods can also help keep you full and satisfied, reducing the likelihood of overeating and snacking on unhealthy foods. This can be especially helpful during intermittent fasting when you're limited in the amount of food you can eat. Foods high in protein include lean meats, poultry, fish, eggs, dairy products, beans, and nuts.

In addition to protein benefits, consuming nutrient-dense foods during your eating periods can provide your body with the essential vitamins, minerals, and other nutrients to function correctly. This helps prevent deficiencies and fuel your body with the best possible nutrition.

It's important to note that not all protein sources are created equal. For example, processed meats and foods high in saturated fat can harm your health, so it's best to choose lean, whole foods that are as close to their natural state as possible.

Healthy fats: While the focus during this diet is often on limiting calorie intake, it's also essential to pay attention to the types of foods you consume during your eating periods. In particular, incorporating healthy fats into your diet can be beneficial for maintaining overall health and wellness during intermittent fasting.

Healthy fats, such as those found in nuts, seeds, avocados, and fatty fish like salmon, play a crucial role in maintaining healthy body weight, supporting brain function, and reducing inflammation. They also provide the body with a slow-burning source of energy that can help you feel full and satisfied for extended periods, reducing the urge to snack and overeat.

In addition to these benefits, healthy fats can also improve the absorption of fat-soluble vitamins, such as A, D, E, and K, essential for maintaining a healthy immune system, good vision, and strong bones. Consuming healthy fats can also help to regulate blood sugar levels, reducing the risk of type 2 diabetes and other chronic health conditions.

It's important to note that not all fats are created equal. While healthy fats are beneficial for the body, unhealthy fats, such as those found in fried foods and processed snacks, can adversely affect health and should be limited in the diet. Trans fats, in particular, should be entirely avoided as they have been linked to heart disease, stroke, and other chronic health conditions.

Fibre-rich foods: Fiber is an essential component of a healthy diet that plays a crucial role in digestive health, weight management, and overall health. Fiber-rich foods, such as whole grains, fruits, vegetables, and legumes, are slowly digested and help to regulate the digestive process, promoting feelings of fullness and reducing the urge to overeat.

In addition to promoting feelings of fullness, fibre supports heart health by reducing cholesterol levels and helping regulate blood sugar levels. This can be especially important during intermittent fasting, as reducing the risk of chronic health conditions is vital to this diet.

Fibre is also crucial for maintaining healthy bowel movements and preventing constipation. This is because fibre acts as a "brush" that cleanses the colon and helps prevent harmful substances buildup. Additionally, fibre helps maintain a healthy gut microbiome, which is essential for overall health and wellness.

Not all fibre is created equal, and it's best to choose fibre-rich foods as close to their natural state as possible. Processed foods and snacks are high in added sugars and low in fibre and should be avoided, as they can harm health.

Hydrating foods: During periods of fasting, the body can become dehydrated, leading to a range of symptoms, including fatigue, headaches, and dry skin. To combat this, it's essential to make sure that you consume enough hydrating foods during your eating periods.

Foods that are high in water content, such as fruits and vegetables, are excellent sources of hydration for the body. These foods are also rich in vitamins, minerals, and antioxidants, which can help to support overall health and wellness. Hydrating foods like watermelon and cucumber can also help regulate body temperature and promote feelings of fullness, reducing the urge to overeat.

In addition to fruits and vegetables, drinking enough water during your eating periods is essential. Staying hydrated helps to flush out toxins, regulate body temperature, and support a healthy immune system. It's also important to choose water as your primary source of hydration, as sugary drinks like soda and juice can adversely affect health.

It's also worth noting that certain medical conditions, such as kidney disease, can impact the body's ability to regulate fluid levels. So if you have any pre-existing health conditions, it's essential to consult with a healthcare professional before starting intermittent fasting to ensure this diet is safe for you.

Low-calorie foods: Low-calorie foods are high in nutrients and low in calories and can help promote feelings of fullness and reduce the urge to overeat. These foods, such as leafy greens, berries, and lean proteins, are rich in vitamins, minerals, and antioxidants and help to support overall health and wellness.

Incorporating low-calorie foods into your diet during intermittent fasting can help to support weight loss and weight management, as they are less likely to contribute to weight gain. Low-calorie foods can also help regulate blood sugar levels, reducing the risk of chronic health conditions like diabetes.

It's essential to choose low-calorie foods that are as close to their natural state as possible. Processed foods and snacks that are high in added sugars and low in nutrients should be avoided, as they can hurt health.

It's also worth noting that calorie needs can vary from person to person and depend on factors like age, sex, and activity level. Suppose you're not sure how many calories you need. In that case, consulting with a healthcare professional or a registered dietitian is a good idea.

Probiotic-rich foods: Probiotics are beneficial bacteria that live in the gut and support digestive health and overall wellness. They play an essential role in regulating the immune system, aiding nutrient absorption, and promoting feelings of fullness.

Incorporating probiotic-rich foods into your diet during intermittent fasting can help to support gut health, reduce inflammation, and improve gut function. These foods, such as yoghurt, kefir, sauerkraut, and kimchi, are rich in probiotics and can help to repopulate the gut with beneficial bacteria.

Choosing probiotic-rich foods that are as close to their natural state as possible is crucial. Processed foods and snacks that are high in added sugars and low in nutrients should be avoided, as they can have a negative impact on gut health.

It's also worth noting that some probiotic-rich foods may contain high amounts of sugar or other unhealthy ingredients. So it's important to read food labels carefully and choose options high in probiotics and low in added sugars and other harmful ingredients.

By incorporating these recommended foods into your intermittent fasting regimen, you can increase the efficiency of your fast and achieve your health and wellness goals. Everyone's nutritional needs and goals are different, so it's essential to listen to your body and adjust your food choices based on your needs and health status.

Maximise Your Intermittent Fasting Success With Hydration

Hydration is crucial in supporting our health, especially during restricted calorie intake. Here's why hydration is especially vital when practising intermittent fasting.

One of the main benefits of intermittent fasting is improved metabolic health. Still, dehydration can cause metabolic disruption and even worsen insulin resistance. Adequate hydration can help the body perform metabolic processes more efficiently and promote overall metabolic health.

Dehydration can also lead to headaches, fatigue, and decreased energy levels. These symptoms can be especially detrimental when trying to fast, making it difficult to maintain and adhere to the fasting schedule. Proper hydration can help keep energy levels up and reduce the risk of headaches and fatigue.

In addition to its metabolic benefits, hydration is also crucial for digestive health. Drinking enough water can help flush out toxins and prevent constipation, which is especially important when following an intermittent fasting protocol. However, dehydration can also cause a build-up of waste in the colon, negatively impacting gut health.

Finally, hydration is essential for mental clarity and cognitive function. When the body is dehydrated, it can lead to feelings of grogginess, confusion, and decreased focus. Maintaining the mental clarity and stress required to adhere to intermittent fasting can make it challenging. Adequate hydration can help improve cognitive function and mental clarity, making staying focused on your fasting goals easier.

What to drink?

Here are some recommended drinks for staying hydrated during intermittent fasting:

Water: Water is the most important and fundamental source of hydration and should be the primary drink of choice during fasting. Aim to drink at least 8-10 glasses of water per day.

Electrolyte-rich drinks: Electrolytes, such as sodium and potassium, are essential for maintaining fluid balance in your body. Try drinking electrolyte-rich drinks like coconut water, sports drinks, or electrolyte tablets in water.

Herbal teas: Herbal teas, such as green tea, ginger tea, and peppermint tea, can help to hydrate you while also providing additional health benefits such as antioxidant support and digestive comfort.

Bone broth: Bone broth is a nourishing and hydrating drink that can help support gut health and boost energy levels during fasting.

Fruit-infused water: Water with lemon, lime, or cucumber, can help to increase your fluid intake while also providing a burst of natural flavour.

Drinking enough fluids during your fasting periods is essential to ensure your fast's success and efficiency. Listen to your body and drink fluids to avoid dehydration and feel your best. Remember, drinking fluids should be a part of your overall healthy eating plan and accompanied by a balanced diet and regular physical activity.

Boost Intermittent Fasting With Supplements and Vitamins

Vitamins and supplements are crucial in supporting our health and wellness, especially during Intermittent fasting, where caloric intake is limited. Here is a more in-depth overview of some of the most essential vitamins and supplements for Intermittent fasting:

Vitamin D: Vitamin D is a fat-soluble vitamin necessary for bone health, immune function, and maintaining a healthy mood.

It is also known as the "sunshine vitamin", as it is produced in our bodies when our skin is exposed to sunlight. However, many people do not get enough vitamin D from sun exposure alone and may need to supplement their diet. A daily dose of 1000-4000 IU is recommended for adults. Too much vitamin D can be toxic, so it is essential to talk to a healthcare professional before starting a supplement regimen.

B-Vitamins: B-vitamins are a group of water-soluble vitamins that play a crucial role in energy production, nervous system function, and cell metabolism. B1 (thiamine), B2 (riboflavin), B6 (pyridoxine), and B12 (cobalamin) are the most critical B vitamins for Intermittent Fasters. Therefore, a daily dose of 50-100 mg of B-complex vitamins is recommended. It is important to note that B vitamins are not stored in our bodies and must be replenished daily through our diet or supplements.

Magnesium: Magnesium is an essential mineral for muscle function, healthy bones, and the nervous system. It also plays a role in energy production and protein synthesis. A daily dose of 300-400 mg is recommended for adults. However, it is important to note that too much magnesium can cause digestive discomfort and other side effects, so talking to a healthcare professional before starting a supplement regimen is essential.

Omega-3 fatty acids: Omega-3 fatty acids are polyunsaturated fats essential for heart health, brain function, and reducing inflammation. They can be found in fatty fish such as salmon and mackerel, as well as in plant-based sources like flaxseed and chia seeds. A daily dose of 1000-2000 mg is recommended for adults. However, it is essential to note that too much omega-3 can increase the risk of bleeding, so it is critical to talk to a healthcare professional before starting a supplement regimen.

Probiotics: Probiotics are live microorganisms that support gut health and healthy digestion. They can be found in fermented foods like yoghurt, kefir, and sauerkraut, as well as in supplements. A daily dose of 10-20 billion CFUs (colony-forming units) is recommended for adults. However, it is essential to note that probiotics can interact with some medications, so talking to a healthcare professional before starting a supplement regimen is vital.

Suppose you're interested in improving your gut health. In that case, probiotic supplements like DuoTrim can be a helpful addition to a balanced diet and lifestyle. DuoTrim contains a unique blend of probiotics and prebiotics that may help support digestive health and overall well-being. In addition, this supplement also promotes weight loss. You can purchase the product through the following QR code:

Fiber: Fiber is an important component of a healthy diet and is important for healthy digestion and satiety. It can be found in foods like whole grains, fruits, and vegetables. A daily dose of 25-30 grams is recommended for adults. It is important to note that increasing fiber intake too quickly can cause digestive discomfort, so it is important to increase fiber intake gradually.

It is important to remember that supplements should be used to complement a balanced diet and regular physical activity, not as a substitute. Talk to a healthcare professional before starting any supplement regimen to ensure the right dosages and to avoid any potential interactions with medications or health conditions.

5 Surprising Tips for a Perfect Blend of Intermittent Fasting and a Balanced Diet

Incorporating Intermittent Fasting (IF) into a balanced diet can provide numerous health benefits, but it's essential to do it correctly. Here are the top 6 tips to help you make the most of your IF journey:

Choose the right IF plan: The proper Intermittent Fasting (IF) plan is crucial for achieving your health and wellness goals. With so many different methods, it's essential to understand the various options and find the one that works best for you.

The first step in choosing the right IF plan is to assess your goals. For example, are you looking to lose weight, improve your overall health, or increase your athletic performance? In addition, different IF plans are designed to meet other goals, so finding the one that aligns with your needs is crucial.

Another vital factor to consider is your lifestyle and schedule. For example, some IF plans require you to fast for extended periods, while others allow shorter fasting windows. Choosing a plan that fits your schedule and will enable you to stick to it in the long term is essential.

Finally, listening to your body and choosing a plan you feel comfortable with is essential. For example, some people may feel fatigued or sluggish during extended fasting periods, while others may feel energised and focused. The right IF plan is the one that works best for your body and allows you to reach your goals.

Plan your meals: Planning your meals in Intermittent Fasting (IF) is critical to making this powerful tool a successful part of your lifestyle. By planning your meals in advance, you can ensure that you get the proper nutrients and fuel your body correctly during your feeding windows.

The first step in meal planning for IF is to assess your nutritional needs. Ensure you're eating a balanced diet with plenty of fruits and vegetables, lean proteins, healthy fats, and whole grains. This will help you feel full and satisfied during your feeding windows and support your overall health.

Next, consider the timing of your meals. Ensure you regularly eat during your feeding windows to maintain stable blood sugar levels and prevent overeating. You may also want to consider prepping your meals in advance to save time and reduce stress during the day.

Finally, be flexible and adaptable. Don't be afraid to change your meal plan as you go along based on how you're feeling and what your body needs. The key is to listen to your body and make adjustments to ensure you're getting the most out of your IF experience.

In conclusion, planning your meals in IF is essential in making this powerful tool a successful part of your lifestyle. By assessing your nutritional needs, timing your meals, and being flexible, you can ensure you're getting the most out of your fasting experience and on the path to optimal health and wellness.

Hydrate: Staying hydrated is crucial for good health, regardless of whether or not you're practising intermittent fasting. It's even more critical to ensure you get enough fluid to support your body's essential functions when you fast.

During a fast, your body is in a state of dehydration. This is because when you don't eat, your body cannot replenish the fluids lost through normal bodily processes like sweating and urination. If you're not careful, this can lead to many health problems, including headaches, fatigue, and even kidney damage.

In addition to these general health risks, dehydration can impact your fasting experience. For example, if you're dehydrated, you may feel fatigued, lightheaded, or experience other symptoms that can make it challenging to stick to your fasting schedule.

The good news is that it's easy to stay hydrated, even when fasting. Simply drink plenty of water and other drinks recommended over the book throughout the day. Some people also find it helpful to drink a glass of water before bed, which can help them stay hydrated overnight.

In conclusion, hydration is crucial to any healthy diet and lifestyle. Still, it's especially important when you're practising intermittent fasting. By consciously staying hydrated, you'll experience all the benefits of fasting while minimizing the risks associated with dehydration.

Listen to your body: Intermittent fasting has gained popularity as a way to improve health and manage weight. However, it's important to remember that what works for one person may not work for another. That's why listening to your body and making adjustments as needed is crucial. Intermittent fasting is not a one-size-fits-all approach to health and wellness.

Your body will give you signals about what it needs and what it can handle. For example, suppose you are feeling weak, fatigued, or starving during fasting. In that case, it may indicate that your body is not well-suited to that approach. On the other hand, if you feel energized, clear-headed, and focused during your fasting periods, it may be a sign that your body is responding well to the approach.

Ultimately, the most important thing is listening to your body and adjusting as needed. If you find that one approach is not working for you, don't be afraid to try a different approach or to make changes to your diet and lifestyle to support your overall health and well-being. Intermittent fasting can be a valuable tool, but it's essential to approach it cautiously and always prioritize your health and well-being.

Avoid overeating during feeding windows: Intermittent fasting can be a powerful tool for improving health and managing weight, but it's important to be mindful of how you approach your feeding windows. While it can be tempting to eat as much as possible during these periods, overeating can undo many of the benefits of fasting and lead to weight gain, digestive problems, and other health issues.

During a feeding window, focusing on eating a balanced diet rich in nutrients, fibre, and healthy fats is essential. This means choosing whole, unprocessed foods whenever possible and avoiding highly processed and sugary foods that can disrupt blood sugar levels and contribute to weight gain.

In addition to focusing on quality, paying attention to portion sizes is essential. Overeating during your feeding windows can lead to weight gain and other health problems, so it's essential to be mindful of how much you're eating and to stop when you feel full.

If you're having trouble controlling your portions, a few strategies can help. For example, eating slowly and taking breaks during your meal can help you tune in to your body's hunger and fullness signals while using smaller plates and bowls can help you control portions more effectively.

In conclusion, avoiding overeating during your feeding windows is integral to making intermittent fasting a successful part of your lifestyle. By focusing on quality and portion control, you can ensure you're getting the most out of your fasting experience and on the path to optimal health and wellness.

Fueling Your Body Right: The Importance of Your First Meal After Intermittent Fasting

The first meal after breaking a fast is crucial because it's when your body is the most receptive to nutrients. Think of it like a sponge that's been wrung out and is now ready to soak up all the goodness you can give it. Your digestive system has been in a resting state and is now primed to receive food. When planning your first meal after breaking the fast, it's important to consider these various food groups and create a balanced meal that incorporates healthy protein, fats, and carbohydrates.

One great option for a healthy protein source is lean meat, such as chicken or turkey. Another excellent choice is cod, which is low in fat and high in protein. This type of protein can help to build and repair muscle, which is important for overall health and fitness.

Healthy fats are also an important component of a well-rounded meal. Avocado is an excellent source of healthy fat, and can be added to salads, smoothies, or eaten on its own. Coconut water is another great option, providing both hydration and essential electrolytes.

Unprocessed carbohydrates are also an important component of a healthy meal. Quinoa is a high-protein, gluten-free grain that can be used as a base for salads or as a side dish. Blackberries are a great source of antioxidants and can be added to smoothies or eaten on their own. Sweet potatoes are a great source of fiber and can be roasted or baked as a side dish.

Finally, vegetables and squash are excellent sources of vitamins and minerals. Roasting or grilling vegetables can bring out their natural flavors, and adding spices or herbs can provide additional health benefits. Squash is a versatile vegetable that can be roasted, grilled, or used in soups and stews.

What You Should Avoid on Your Intermittent Fasting Journey

Intermittent fasting can effectively improve your health and reach your weight loss goals, but it's not always easy to navigate. One of the most important factors to consider is your intake of sugar and alcohol during fasting. While it may be tempting to indulge in your favourite treats, it can have a negative impact on the benefits of fasting.

When you consume sugar or alcohol, it can interfere with the body's natural fasting process. This can cause disruptions to insulin levels, leading to a decrease in fat burning and a spike in blood glucose levels. Alcohol can also cause dehydration, which can make fasting more challenging and disrupt sleep, a critical factor in the overall benefits of fasting.

So, how can you limit your sugar and alcohol intake during fasting? The key is to be mindful of your consumption and make small changes to your diet. Try to replace sugary or alcoholic drinks with water, herbal tea, or black coffee, which can keep you hydrated and alert during the fast.

If you find yourself struggling with cravings for sugary or alcoholic drinks, try incorporating healthy snacks and meals during your feeding window. This can include healthy meat proteins like chicken or fish, avocado or coconut oil for healthy fats, and unprocessed carbohydrates like quinoa or sweet potatoes. Vegetables and berries are also great options for fibre and micronutrients.

Making these small changes ensures you're getting the most out of your intermittent fasting journey. So, be mindful of sugar and alcohol intake and incorporate healthier options into your diet. Your body will thank you for it!

Know Your Optimal Calories Intake

To calculate your calorie intake during Intermittent Fasting (IF), consider a few things, including your age, weight, height, activity level, and weight loss goals. Here's a basic outline of how to calculate your calorie needs:

1. Determine your Basal Metabolic Rate (BMR): Your BMR is the number of calories your body needs to function while at rest. You can use an online BMR calculator to determine this number.

2. Adjust for activity level: Once you know your BMR, you need to adjust for your activity level to determine your Total Daily Energy Expenditure (TDEE). You can use a TDEE calculator to do this. https://tdeecalculator.net/

3. Determine your calorie intake during the eating window: Based on your TDEE, determine the number of calories you want to consume during your eating window. If you're trying to lose weight, you must consume fewer calories than your TDEE. If you're trying to maintain weight, you'll want to consume the same calories as your TDEE. If you're trying to gain weight, you must consume more calories than your TDEE.

4. Continue to exercise: Exercising while practising Intermittent Fasting (IF) is an essential part of maximizing the health benefits of this powerful tool. Exercise not only helps to support physical health but also improves mental wellbeing and helps to keep your metabolism running smoothly.

Finding a routine that works for you and your lifestyle is critical for exercise and IF. For some, this may mean engaging in high-intensity interval training during the feeding windows. In contrast, others may prefer more low-impact activities like yoga or walking.

It's important to remember that exercise during IF can also help to regulate blood sugar levels, boost energy, and reduce feelings of fatigue. In addition, regular physical activity can help to reduce stress and promote better sleep, both of which are critical to overall health and wellbeing.

For example, if you're feeling low on energy, you may need to reduce the intensity or frequency of your workouts. On the other hand, if you're feeling energized, you may want to push yourself a bit further to maximize the benefits.

7

— • —

INTERMITTENT FASTING AS A TOOL FOR WEIGHT LOSS

Weight loss is an issue that affects millions of people worldwide. In many cases, individuals who struggle with weight gain and obesity face various health issues, including an increased risk of heart disease, diabetes, and other chronic diseases. For this reason, it is essential to focus on strategies that can help individuals achieve and maintain a healthy weight, such as intermittent fasting.

Intermittent fasting is a dietary approach that involves alternating periods of eating and fasting. This method is believed to be an effective way to reduce calorie intake, which can lead to weight loss. In addition, intermittent fasting has been linked to other health benefits, such as improved insulin sensitivity, lower inflammation, and a reduced risk of chronic disease.

The Importance of Weight Loss in Health

The importance of weight loss in health cannot be overstated. Excess weight can strain the body and increase the risk of several health issues, including diabetes, high blood pressure, heart disease, and stroke. In addition, being overweight can lead to lower self-esteem, depression, and anxiety, affecting an individual's mental and emotional well-being.

Maintaining a healthy weight is an essential part of a healthy lifestyle. A healthy weight can help individuals reduce their risk of chronic diseases, improve their energy levels and mood, and boost their overall quality of life. However, achieving and maintaining a healthy weight can be challenging, especially for individuals who struggle with weight gain and obesity.

Intermittent fasting has become a popular approach to weight loss in recent years. This approach involves cycling between periods of eating and fasting, which can help reduce calorie intake and promote weight loss. In addition, intermittent fasting has been shown to have several other health benefits, including improved insulin sensitivity, reduced inflammation, and a decreased risk of chronic diseases.

One of the reasons why intermittent fasting is believed to be effective for weight loss is that it can help reduce overall calorie intake. Limiting the number of hours an individual can eat makes them naturally more likely to consume fewer calories. For example, an individual who practices the 16/8 method of intermittent fasting will typically eat all their meals during an 8-hour window, from 11 am to 7 pm. This means they will naturally eat fewer calories than eating for 12 or 14 hours a day.

Another way that intermittent fasting may help with weight loss is by reducing insulin resistance. Insulin resistance occurs when the body becomes less responsive to the hormone insulin, which can lead to high blood sugar levels and weight gain. Intermittent fasting has been shown to improve insulin sensitivity, which may help with weight loss and reduce the risk of type 2 diabetes.

Scientific Research on Intermittent Fasting and Weight Loss

Several scientific studies have explored the effectiveness of intermittent fasting for weight loss. For example, in one study, participants who practised intermittent fasting lost more weight than those who followed a traditional calorie-restricted diet. The study found that the participants who followed an irregular fasting plan lost an average of 8 pounds over eight weeks, while those who followed a traditional calorie-restricted diet lost an average of 5.5 pounds.

Another study found that intermittent fasting can lead to decreased body fat and increased muscle mass. The study, which involved overweight men, found that those who practised intermittent fasting lost more body fat and gained more muscle mass than those who followed a traditional calorie-restricted diet.

Most Effective Types of Intermittent Fasting for Weight Loss

There are several different types of intermittent fasting, each with unique benefits and challenges. The most common types of intermittent fasting include 16/8, 5:2, and alternate-day fasting.

The 16/8 method involves fasting for 16 hours and eating all meals within an 8-hour window. This approach is easy to follow and can be incorporated into most lifestyles. The 5:2 method involves eating normally five days a week and limiting calorie intake to 500-600 calories for two non-consecutive days. Finally, alternate-day fasting involves fasting every other day, with calorie intake limited to 500-600 calories on fasting days.

While all types of intermittent fasting can lead to weight loss, the most effective weight loss will depend on an individual's lifestyle, preferences, and goals. It is essential to consult a healthcare professional before starting any new diet or exercise plan.

Weight Loss Plateaus During Intermittent Fasting

One challenge individuals may face while practising intermittent fasting is a weight loss plateau. A weight loss plateau occurs when an individual's weight loss stalls or slows down despite continued efforts to lose weight.

Several factors can contribute to weight loss plateaus, including decreased metabolic rate, reduced calorie deficit, and hormonal changes. Weight loss plateaus can be frustrating, but they are a natural part of weight loss.

Breaking through a weight loss plateau during intermittent fasting requires a multi-faceted approach. However, some strategies that can help individuals break through a weight loss plateau include:

1.   Increase physical activity: Incorporating more exercise into your routine can help boost metabolism and burn more calories.

2.   Change your eating pattern: Switching up your eating pattern can help kickstart weight loss. For example, if you typically practice the 16/8 method, you could switch to alternate-day fasting or the 5:2 method.

3.   Reduce calorie intake: If you have been eating at maintenance or surplus, consider reducing your calorie intake to create a calorie deficit again.

4.   Increase water intake: Drinking more water can help reduce hunger and boost metabolism.

5.   Focus on nutrient-dense foods: Eating foods high in nutrients and low in calories can help you feel full while consuming fewer calories.

Fasting for Weight Loss: How Long Does It Take to See Results?

When it comes to weight loss, many people turn to intermittent fasting as a powerful tool to help shed those extra pounds. However, it's essential to understand that the timeframe for seeing results with intermittent fasting can vary from person to person.

For some individuals, noticeable changes may occur within a few weeks of starting intermittent fasting. These changes can include improved energy levels, reduced cravings, and initial weight loss.

However, it's essential to remember that sustainable weight loss takes time and patience.

The first few weeks of intermittent fasting may primarily involve your body adapting to the new eating pattern. During this time, your metabolism may adjust, and your body may tap into stored fat for energy. However, significant weight loss typically occurs over a more extended period.

Most experts suggest that a consistent and disciplined approach to intermittent fasting, a healthy diet, and regular exercise can lead to steady weight loss throughout 6 to 10 weeks. However, it's important to note that everyone's journey is unique, and factors such as individual metabolism, starting weight, and overall lifestyle habits can influence the pace of weight loss. Remember, the key to success with intermittent fasting is consistency and patience. Finding a fasting schedule that works best for you and your lifestyle is crucial.

Conclusion

In conclusion, weight loss is essential to maintaining good health, and intermittent fasting is a practical approach to achieving and maintaining a healthy weight. Intermittent fasting can lead to weight loss, improved insulin sensitivity, reduced inflammation, and a decreased risk of chronic diseases.

While there is no one-size-fits-all approach to intermittent fasting, finding the suitable method for an individual's lifestyle, preferences, and goals is critical. Additionally, weight loss plateaus are a natural part of the weight loss process, and strategies such as increasing physical activity, changing eating patterns, and reducing calorie intake can help break through them.

Individualized weight loss goals and strategies are essential for long-term success, and it is vital to consult a healthcare professional before starting any new diet or exercise plan. In addition, individuals can achieve sustained weight loss and improved health by practising intermittent fasting and healthy lifestyle changes.

Are you looking for a natural way to boost your weight loss journey? Meet Alpilean, a new supplement making waves in the fitness world. Alpilean is formulated with natural ingredients that help suppress your appetite, boost your energy levels, and boost your metabolism. So, try it out and let Alpilean help you achieve your goals healthily and effectively.

8

---·---

INTERMITTENT FASTING FOR DIFFERENT POPULATIONS

Approaching Intermittent Fasting (IF) requires an individualized approach, considering personal factors such as physical activity level, medical history, and overall health goals. What works for one person may not work for another, and finding a plan that fits your specific needs and lifestyle is key.

For example, some individuals may benefit from more extended fasting periods. In contrast, others may need shorter periods or may even find that fasting is not suitable for them at all. Additionally, the type of food consumed during feeding significantly impacts overall health and wellness. Essential to focus on nutrient-dense, whole foods that support general wellbeing and wellbeing.

To get an increased perception of what suits your specific needs the best, follow the following population categorization.

Intermittent Fasting for Women

Women have unique physiological and hormonal considerations when it comes to fasting, and it's vital to approach IF in a way that considers these factors.

Women have a higher likelihood of experiencing symptoms such as low energy, mood swings, and disrupted sleep when fasting, as changes in hormone levels can impact the body's ability to regulate hunger and energy levels. Some women may also experience menstrual irregularities or hormonal imbalances when fasting, which can be concerning for some.

Women must choose a fasting plan that fits their needs and goals. For example, shorter fasting or a more gradual approach may be more appropriate for some women. In comparison, others may benefit from more extended fasting periods. It's also essential to ensure adequate amounts of nutrients are consumed during feeding windows and monitor how the body responds to fasting.

In conclusion, women can benefit from incorporating intermittent fasting into their diet. Still, they must consider the unique characteristics of their bodies. By following these tips, women can maximize the benefits of intermittent fasting and achieve their health and wellness goals.

Women Over 50

As women age and enter their 50s and beyond, they experience a range of changes in their bodies that can significantly impact their approach to Intermittent Fasting (IF). One of the most significant changes is hormonal, as menopause and other hormonal shifts can affect metabolism and energy levels.

When it comes to IF, these changes can mean that women over 50 must approach fasting in a more mindful and tailored way. For example, they may need to limit their fasting periods to shorter ones, as hormonal changes can affect their ability to regulate hunger and energy levels. Additionally, women over 50 may need to be mindful of their nutrient intake during feeding windows, as their metabolism may not be as efficient at processing certain foods.

Another factor to consider is the impact of metabolic changes on weight management, as women over 50 may experience a slowdown in metabolism, making it more challenging to manage their weight. However, by approaching IF in a way that supports overall health and wellness, women over 50 can help mitigate these challenges and get the most out of their experience.

Intermittent Fasting for Men

Intermittent fasting can be a practical approach to health and wellness for men. Still, it's essential to consider the unique characteristics of the male body when designing a fasting plan. For example, men generally have higher muscle mass and lower body fat than women, affecting their metabolism. Additionally, hormonal changes that occur as men age can also play a role in the efficacy of IF.

To maximize the benefits of IF for men, choosing a fasting plan that considers these characteristics is essential. A 16/8 fasting schedule can be an excellent place to start, and the fasting period can be gradually extended if desired. It's also important to focus on nutrient-dense foods during the eating window, such as high-quality protein, fibre-rich vegetables, and healthy fats.

Staying hydrated is vital for men during their fasting period, as it can help maintain energy levels and support overall health. Regular exercise is also crucial for men during IF, as it can help increase muscle mass and improve metabolism.

Athletes and Active Individuals

Intermittent fasting has become a popular diet approach for athletes and active individuals who are looking to improve their performance and overall health. However, it's important to note that this diet may not be suitable for everyone, and athletes must take into account their unique energy needs and athletic goals before adopting an intermittent fasting plan.

For athletes who choose to incorporate intermittent fasting into their routine, it's crucial to select a fasting plan that aligns with their daily activities and allows for sufficient energy during intense training sessions. This requires careful planning and preparation, such as scheduling workouts during the eating window or adjusting the fasting schedule to accommodate training sessions.

On a day-to-day basis, athletes can cope with intermittent fasting by making sure to consume nutrient-dense, calorie-rich foods during the eating window. A balanced diet that includes high-quality protein, complex carbohydrates, fiber-rich vegetables, and healthy fats can help support recovery and promote overall health.

Hydration is also vital for athletes during fasting periods, as it can help maintain energy levels and support overall health. It's recommended that athletes drink plenty of water and electrolyte-rich beverages throughout the day to stay hydrated and prevent dehydration.

Lastly, athletes must listen to their bodies and adjust their fasting approach accordingly. If they experience fatigue or adverse side effects, they may need to reconsider their plan and make modifications to ensure their unique energy needs are being met. Overall, intermittent fasting can be a useful tool for athletes and active individuals, but it must be approached with caution and careful consideration.

Muscle Gains

Intermittent fasting is often associated with weight loss, but did you know that it can also contribute to muscle gain? While it may seem counterintuitive to fast when building muscle, it can be a powerful tool in your arsenal.

One way intermittent fasting can contribute to muscle gain is by increasing human growth hormone (HGH) production. HGH is a hormone that stimulates muscle growth and repair, and intermittent fasting has been shown to increase its production by up to 5 times. This increase in HGH can lead to greater muscle mass and strength gains over time.

Intermittent fasting also promotes fat loss while preserving muscle mass. This is because when you fast, your body switches from burning glucose (sugar) for energy to burning fat instead. This can help reduce overall body fat percentage, making your muscles more visible and defined.

In addition, intermittent fasting has been shown to improve insulin sensitivity, which can help your body better utilize nutrients from the food you eat. This can lead to better muscle growth and recovery after workouts.

Of course, it's important to remember that building muscle requires consistent strength training and adequate protein intake.

9

— ● —

INTERMITTENT FASTING FOR RISK POPULATIONS

I ntermittent fasting has become a popular diet trend in recent years due to its potential health benefits. However, certain groups of people, known as risk populations, may require extra caution when considering this type of diet. Risk populations include pregnant and breastfeeding women, children, and individuals with certain medical conditions.

While intermittent fasting may be feasible for some risk populations, it is essential to seek guidance from a healthcare professional before starting.

In this chapter, we will discuss the potential benefits and risks of intermittent fasting for risk populations and provide guidance on how to approach this type of diet according to your needs

Pregnant and Breastfeeding Women

Pregnancy and breastfeeding are essential stages in a woman's life, and it's vital to approach Intermittent Fasting (IF) in a way that supports both the health of the mother and the growing baby.

Pregnant women should be cautious when considering IF, as their bodies undergo significant changes and have increased nutritional needs. Pregnant women require a balanced and consistent intake of nutrients to support the growth and development of their babies, and fasting could limit their intake of essential nutrients. Additionally, the fluctuations in blood sugar levels that can occur during IF can be problematic for pregnant women, as this can affect the developing fetus. The following list consists of tips for the success of IF among pregnant women. These top 5 tips are essential and should be considered before starting IF.

· Consult a doctor or a registered dietitian before starting any fasting plan to ensure it's safe and appropriate for their needs. Pregnant women have unique nutritional deficiencies, and it's essential to make sure that any fasting plan is safe and suitable for their individual needs.

· Incorporate nutrient-dense foods in their diet during feeding windows. This can include leafy greens, lean proteins, whole grains, and healthy fats. These foods provide essential vitamins and minerals necessary for maintaining a healthy pregnancy.

· Stay hydrated throughout the day, as dehydration can lead to headaches, fatigue, and other symptoms. Drinking plenty of water, herbal teas, and other fluids can help keep the body hydrated and support a healthy pregnancy.

· Avoid skipping meals or limiting food intake during feeding windows, as this can lead to nutrient deficiencies and impact the health of both the mother and the baby. Instead, eating enough calories to maintain energy levels and support a healthy pregnancy is essential.

· Consider alternative fasting methods, such as time-restricted eating or moderate calorie restriction, that are less restrictive and easier to stick to during pregnancy. It's crucial to approach IF in a way that supports a healthy pregnancy and the baby's health.

Breastfeeding is an essential part of motherhood, providing vital nutrients to nourish and support a growing baby. But did you know that fasting while breastfeeding can have a significant impact on the quality and quantity of milk produced? As a breastfeeding mother, your top priority is to maintain a healthy milk supply and ensure that your baby receives the essential nutrients they need for optimal growth and development.

Fasting can be tempting, especially when trying to shed post-pregnancy pounds. However, it's critical to consider the potential consequences of fasting while breastfeeding. Research has shown that fasting can reduce the amount and quality of milk produced, which can negatively impact your baby's health and development.

The good news is that there are ways for breastfeeding mothers to incorporate intermittent fasting safely into their daily routine. The key is to focus on consuming nutrient-dense foods that provide essential vitamins and minerals necessary for maintaining healthy milk production. Foods like leafy greens, lean proteins, whole grains, and healthy fats should be incorporated into your diet during feeding windows.

It's also crucial for breastfeeding women to stay hydrated throughout the day, as dehydration can affect milk production and lead to headaches and fatigue. Drinking plenty of water, herbal teas, and other fluids can help keep your body hydrated and support milk production.

Furthermore, it's essential to avoid skipping meals or limiting food intake during feeding windows. Doing so can lead to nutrient deficiencies and impact milk production. Instead, consuming enough calories is vital to maintain energy levels and support milk production.

In summary, while intermittent fasting can be a useful tool for weight loss and overall health, it's essential to approach it safely as a breastfeeding mother. By focusing on nutrient-dense foods, staying hydrated, and consuming enough calories, you can support healthy milk production while still reaping the benefits of intermittent fasting.

Intermittent Fasting for Children

Children require adequate nutrition to support their growth and development. Intermittent fasting may lead to insufficient essential nutrients such as protein, vitamins, and minerals, negatively impacting a child's health.

Furthermore, children are still developing their relationship with food. They may not have the emotional maturity to handle the restrictions and potential hunger associated with fasting. Intermittent fasting could lead to disordered eating behaviours or a negative body image in some children.

Parents must consult with a healthcare professional before considering implementing intermittent fasting for their children. A qualified healthcare provider can evaluate the child's nutritional needs, overall health, and growth patterns to determine if intermittent fasting is appropriate.

Intermittent Fasting for Individuals With Medical Conditions

Intermittent fasting can benefit individuals with certain medical conditions. Still, it is crucial to approach it with caution and proper planning. Here are a few common medical conditions to consider:

Diabetes: If you have diabetes, Intermittent Fasting (IF) can be a bit more complicated. People with diabetes need to be particularly mindful of their blood sugar levels and insulin sensitivity, which can be affected by the timing and frequency of meals.

For individuals with type 1 diabetes, monitor blood glucose levels closely and adjust insulin doses as needed. Skipping meals or going without food for extended periods can be dangerous for those with type 1 diabetes and may lead to hypoglycaemia.

For individuals with type 2 diabetes, Intermittent Fasting may be beneficial in managing blood glucose levels. IF has been shown to improve insulin sensitivity and can help regulate glucose levels. Still, working with a healthcare professional is vital to ensure it's the right approach for you.

For individuals with type 3 diabetes, intermittent fasting has been shown to have potential benefits for individuals with type 3 diabetes. By limiting the times when they consume calories, it can help improve insulin sensitivity and reduce blood sugar levels.

However, it is crucial for individuals with type 3 diabetes to consult with a medical professional before starting an intermittent fasting regimen. A doctor or a nutritionist can help assess their individual situation, recommend a suitable approach, and monitor their progress.

It's essential to remember that everyone's diabetes is different, and what works for one person may not work for another.

Low blood pressure: Low blood pressure, also known as hypotension, is a medical condition where a person has a lower-than-normal blood pressure reading. For individuals with low blood pressure, it is crucial to approach intermittent fasting with caution and under the guidance of a healthcare professional. Intermittent fasting may affect blood pressure levels and lead to dizziness, fainting, or weakness if not done correctly.

For individuals with low blood pressure, avoiding extreme fasting periods and instead opting for shorter fasting windows is recommended. They should also ensure to consume enough fluids during their feeding windows, as dehydration can worsen symptoms of low blood pressure. Additionally, they should consume balanced meals and snacks and include plenty of nutrients to maintain proper blood pressure levels.

Eating Disorders: Eating disorders are complex mental health conditions that involve a range of abnormal behaviours and attitudes related to food and weight. These disorders can have severe consequences for physical health and significantly affect an individual's psychological wellbeing. Intermittent fasting, which involves periodic periods of restricted food intake, may be especially concerning for individuals with a history of eating disorders.

For those with an eating disorder, such as anorexia or bulimia, fasting or restricting food intake can trigger harmful thoughts and behaviours. The focus on food and weight can be intense, leading to an increased risk of relapse or exacerbation of symptoms.

It is vital for individuals with a history of eating disorders to seek the guidance of a mental health professional and registered dietitian before starting any type of fasting regimen. Then, they can work together to create a safe and effective plan that considers the individual's unique needs and challenges. This may include incorporating regular meals, balanced nutrition, and strategies to manage disordered thoughts and behaviours related to food and weight.

Gastrointestinal issues: Gastrointestinal issues, such as irritable bowel syndrome (IBS), inflammatory bowel disease (IBD), and acid reflux, can significantly impact how an individual approaches intermittent fasting.

Sometimes, skipping meals or fasting long periods can exacerbate symptoms and cause discomfort. Individuals with gastrointestinal issues need to work closely with a healthcare professional to develop a safe and effective approach to intermittent fasting. This may involve modifications to the type of food consumed during feeding windows, the length of fasting periods, and the frequency. For example, incorporating high-fibre, low-fat foods and avoiding trigger foods during feeding windows can help alleviate symptoms and improve overall gut health.

It may also be necessary to break fasts with smaller, more frequent meals instead of large, heavy meals. In some cases, it may be advised to avoid intermittent fasting altogether. The approach to intermittent fasting for individuals with gastrointestinal issues will vary based on the specific condition and the severity of symptoms, so it is vital to seek individualized guidance.

Kidney issues: Intermittent fasting can be challenging for individuals with kidney issues, as they need to maintain a balanced intake of fluids and electrolytes. Here are some practical tips:

· Monitor fluid and electrolyte levels: IF can result in dehydration, harming individuals with kidney problems. They should drink enough water and monitor their fluid levels, especially during fasting.

· Choose the correct type of IF: People with kidney problems may want to avoid long fasting periods and choose a more moderate form of IF.

· Avoid fasting during a flare-up: People with kidney problems may experience a flare-up during stress or illness. They should avoid fasting and stick to their regular eating habits during such times.

Liver Issues: Intermittent fasting can affect people with liver issues differently, as it may place additional stress on the liver. Here are some practical tips:

· Choose the correct type of IF: People with liver problems may want to avoid long fasting periods and choose a more moderate form of IF.

· Monitor liver function: People with liver problems should regularly monitor their liver function tests and report any changes to their doctor.

· Avoid fasting during a flare-up: People with liver problems may experience a flare-up during stress or illness. They should avoid fasting and stick to their regular eating habits during such times.

It's crucial to approach intermittent fasting with a positive mindset and determination. It may require more planning and preparation, but with the right mindset, you can successfully incorporate fasting into your lifestyle and see significant improvements in your health.

It's important to keep in mind that intermittent fasting is not a one-size-fits-all method. Every individual has unique needs and considerations, and it's essential to tailor the fasting plan to your specific medical condition. With careful planning, support from healthcare professionals, and a positive attitude, you can successfully incorporate intermittent fasting into your life and achieve your health goals.

10

20 Mouth-Watering Meal Ideas to Elevate Your Intermittent Fasting Experience

I ncorporating Intermittent Fasting into your daily routine can be a bit daunting at first, especially when it comes to meal planning. But with a little bit of creativity, you can easily make satisfying and nutritious meals that will not only help you stick to your fasting schedule but also make the experience enjoyable. In this chapter, we have compiled 20 delicious meal ideas that will help you make the most of your Intermittent Fasting journey. Whether you are a beginner or a seasoned practitioner, you are sure to find some inspiration here. So sit back, grab a notebook, and get ready to plan some mouth-watering meals that will make your fasting experience a breeze.

The meal ideas will be splited into four different categories, based on the type of Intermittent Fasting method you prefer.

16/8 method:

Day 1:

Breakfast: Whole grain toast with avocado and a fried egg. (400 calories)

Lunch: Grilled chicken breast with mixed veggies and a side of quinoa. (450 calories)

Dinner: Baked salmon with roasted sweet potatoes and a green salad. (450 calories)

Day 2:

Breakfast: Greek yogurt with mixed berries and a sprinkle of granola. (350 calories)

Lunch: Turkey and cheese wrap with a side of fruit. (400 calories)

Dinner: Veggie stir fry with tofu and brown rice. (450 calories)

Day 3:

Breakfast: Oatmeal with almond milk, cinnamon and sliced almonds. (400 calories)

Lunch: Chickpea salad with mixed greens and a side of whole grain crackers. (400 calories)

Dinner: Grilled steak with roasted vegetables and a baked potato. (500 calories)

Day 4:

Breakfast: Scrambled eggs with whole grain toast and a side of fruit. (400 calories)

Lunch: Grilled shrimp with mixed veggies and a side of brown rice. (450 calories)

Dinner: Lentil soup with a mixed greens salad and whole grain bread. (450 calories)

Day 5:

Breakfast: Peanut butter and banana smoothie. (400 calories)

Lunch: Veggie burger with mixed greens and a side of sweet potato fries. (450 calories)

Dinner: Grilled chicken breast with mixed veggies and a side of quinoa. (450 calories)

5:2 Diet:

Day 1:

Breakfast: 1 hard-boiled egg, 1 small whole grain toast with avocado, 1 cup of low-fat yogurt (Total calories: 250)

Lunch: Grilled chicken breast (3 oz), mixed greens salad with tomato, cucumber, and lemon dressing (Total calories: 200)

Dinner: Steamed salmon (3 oz) with roasted vegetables (zucchini, bell peppers, and mushrooms) (Total calories: 200)

Day 2:

Breakfast: Greek yogurt with mixed berries, 1 piece of whole grain toast with almond butter, 1 boiled egg (Total calories: 300)

Lunch: Lentil soup with mixed veggies, 1 whole grain roll (Total calories: 250)

Dinner: Grilled lean steak (3 oz) with quinoa and steamed broccoli (Total calories: 250)

Day 3:

Breakfast: Scrambled eggs with chopped veggies (tomatoes, mushrooms, and bell peppers), 1 piece of whole grain toast (Total calories: 250)

Lunch: Grilled chicken salad (lettuce, tomatoes, cucumber, and carrots) with vinaigrette dressing (Total calories: 200)

Dinner: Grilled shrimp (4 oz) with brown rice and steamed asparagus (Total calories: 250)

Day 4:

Breakfast: Chia seed pudding with mixed nuts and berries (Total calories: 300)

Lunch: Tuna salad (lettuce, tomato, and cucumber) with whole grain crackers (Total calories: 250)

Dinner: Grilled pork tenderloin (3 oz) with sweet potato and steamed green beans (Total calories: 250)

Day 5:

Breakfast: Peanut butter and banana smoothie (Total calories: 300)

Lunch: Grilled chicken and vegetable skewers (zucchini, bell peppers, and onions) (Total calories: 200)

Dinner: Baked cod (3 oz) with quinoa and roasted carrots (Total calories: 200)

These meal plans aim to provide healthy and delicious options while following the 5:2 diet intermittent fasting method.

Alternate-day Fasting:

Day 1 (Fasting Day):

Breakfast: Black coffee or tea with lemon, cinnamon, and a touch of honey.

Lunch: Chicken broth with grated ginger, garlic, and turmeric.

Dinner: Grilled salmon with roasted vegetables and a side of quinoa.

Snack: Fresh fruit salad with a drizzle of honey and lemon juice.

Total Caloric Intake: Approximately 500 calories.

Day 2 (Feeding Day):

Breakfast: Avocado and egg toast with a side of cherry tomatoes.

Lunch: Grilled chicken breast with sweet potato wedges and steamed broccoli.

Dinner: Whole wheat spaghetti with meat sauce and a side of garlic bread.

Snacks: Yogurt with fresh berries and a handful of almonds.

Total Caloric Intake: Approximately 1500 calories.

Day 3 (Fasting Day):

Breakfast: Green tea with lemon and honey.

Lunch: Clear vegetable soup with a side of whole grain crackers.

Dinner: Grilled shrimp with roasted asparagus and a side of brown rice.

Snack: Apple slices with almond butter.

Total Caloric Intake: Approximately 500 calories.

Day 4 (Feeding Day):

Breakfast: Greek yogurt with granola and fresh fruit.

Lunch: Grilled turkey burger with a side of sweet potato fries.

Dinner: Stuffed bell peppers with quinoa, cheese, and tomato sauce.

Snack: Rice crackers with hummus and carrot sticks.

Total Caloric Intake: Approximately 1500 calories.

Day 5 (Fasting Day):

Breakfast: Chia seed pudding with almond milk and fresh berries.

Lunch: Minestrone soup with a side of whole grain bread.

Dinner: Grilled steak with roasted Brussels sprouts and a side of mashed sweet potatoes.

Snack: Freshly squeezed juice with ginger and turmeric.

Total Caloric Intake: Approximately 500 calories.

Day 6 (Feeding Day):

Breakfast: Scrambled eggs with whole grain toast and spinach.

Lunch: Grilled chicken fajitas with a side of corn on the cob.

Dinner: Baked salmon with roasted vegetables and a side of brown rice.

Snack: Dark chocolate with almonds.

Total Caloric Intake: Approximately 1500 calories.

Day 7 (Fasting Day):

Breakfast: Herbal tea with lemon and honey.

Lunch: Vegetable stir-fry with tofu and a side of brown rice.

Dinner: Grilled lamb chops with roasted root vegetables.

Snack: Fresh fruit smoothie with almond milk and honey.

Total Caloric Intake: Approximately 500 calories.

24 Hour Fasting Method:

Day 1:

Breakfast: Greek yogurt with mixed berries and a drizzle of honey (400 calories)

Lunch: Grilled chicken breast with roasted vegetables (400 calories)

Dinner: Lentil soup with crusty bread (500 calories)

Snack: Apple slices with almond butter (200 calories)

Total: 1500 calories

Day 3:

Breakfast: Veggie omelette with mushrooms, spinach and feta cheese (400 calories)

Lunch: Tuna salad with cherry tomatoes, cucumber and light dressing (400 calories)

Dinner: Baked salmon with quinoa and steamed broccoli (500 calories)

Snack: Carrot sticks with hummus (200 calories)

Total: 1500 calories

Day 5:

Breakfast: Peanut butter banana smoothie (400 calories)

Lunch: Grilled chicken with sweet potato wedges (400 calories)

Dinner: Stuffed bell peppers with quinoa, black beans and salsa (500 calories)

Snack: Rice crackers with avocado dip (200 calories)

Total: 1500 calories

Day 7:

Breakfast: Oatmeal with almond milk, cinnamon and raisins (400 calories)

Lunch: Turkey sandwich with whole grain bread, lettuce and tomato (400 calories)

Dinner: Baked chicken with mixed veggies and brown rice (500 calories)

Snack: Popcorn (200 calories)

Total: 1500 calories

As you embark on your intermittent fasting journey, it's essential to consider how your age affects your calorie needs. As we age, our metabolism slows down, meaning we require fewer calories to sustain our bodies. Your body's needs can be met while still sticking to your fasting schedule by adjusting your calorie intake. Similarly, weight is a critical factor in determining calorie needs during intermittent fasting. If you're carrying excess weight, your body requires more calories to maintain that weight. On the other hand, if you're underweight, you may need to increase your calorie intake to meet your body's requirements. Understanding your ideal weight and adjusting your calorie intake accordingly can help you achieve your weight loss goals and improve your overall health.

Other specifications, such as height and activity level, are also essential when determining your calorie needs during intermittent fasting. Taller individuals or those who engage in high levels of physical activity will require more calories to sustain their bodies during fasting. By considering your age, weight, and other specifications when approaching intermittent fasting, you can tailor your fasting plan to meet your body's unique needs.

11

— • —

CONCLUSION

In conclusion, "The Ultimate Guide to Intermittent Fasting for Beginners" provides a comprehensive and approachable introduction to this powerful health and wellness tool. With a focus on the science behind Intermittent Fasting and its many benefits, this guide is a valuable resource for anyone looking to learn more about this increasingly popular practice.

From the different methods of Intermittent Fasting to practical tips for getting started, this guide covers everything you need to know to make the most of your Intermittent Fasting experience. Whether you're new to Intermittent Fasting or looking to refine your existing practice, the information and insights in this guide will help you achieve your health and wellness goals.

In addition to its comprehensive information, this guide also includes delicious meal ideas to elevate your Intermittent Fasting experience, making it easier and more enjoyable to stick to your fasting regimen. With its approachable and engaging tone, "The

Ultimate Guide to Intermittent Fasting for Beginners" is the perfect tool for anyone looking to explore the power of Intermittent Fasting for their own health and wellness journey.

Ultimately, with the right approach and mindset, intermittent fasting can be a sustainable and effective way to improve your overall health and wellbeing. So, take the information and tips provided in this guide, and start exploring the transformative power of intermittent fasting today!

Special Bonus

If you're on a journey to optimal health and weight loss, you're probably aware of the importance of a balanced diet and regular exercise. But what about dessert? We crave something sweet but often feel guilty indulging in our favourite treats. That's where our FREE guide comes in. The Top 7 Delicious Fat Burning Desserts That No Nutritionist Would Dare Tell You is the perfect companion to your intermittent fasting journey. It lets you satisfy your sweet tooth without compromising your weight loss progress. So why not take advantage of this opportunity and download our guide for FREE? Your taste buds and your waistline will thank you.

Printed in Great Britain
by Amazon